# ELEVATE YOUR LIFE: A GUIDE TO DAILY HEALTHY LIVING HABITS

## DAILY HEALTH TIPS & GOALS

HABIB ZAKARI MOHAMMED

ISBN: 9798876211996

# DEDICATION

To my wife Habeebah, for all her support!

# CONTENTS

## Understanding Sleep: Nurturing Your Body's Reset Button

*Introduction:* Sleep isn't just a nightly routine; it's a fundamental pillar of overall health. In this section, we delve into the intricate relationship between sleep and well-being, unlocking the secrets behind quality rest and its profound impact on your physical and mental vitality.

**The Sleep-Health Connection:** *The Brain's Nightly Cleanup:* During sleep, your brain undergoes a meticulous cleaning process, flushing out toxins accumulated during the day. This supports cognitive function, memory consolidation, and emotional regulation.
*Cognitive and Emotional Resilience:* Quality sleep fosters better decision-making, emotional resilience, and a positive outlook. Understanding this connection emphasizes the pivotal role of sleep in mental health.

**Establishing a Consistent Sleep Schedule:** *The Power of Routine:* Your body thrives on consistency. Establishing a regular sleep schedule helps regulate your internal clock, making it easier to fall asleep and wake up naturally.
*Nighttime Rituals:* Incorporating calming rituals before bedtime signals to your body that it's time to wind down. This might include activities like reading, gentle stretching, or practicing relaxation techniques.

**Creating a Relaxing Bedtime Routine:** *Limiting Stimulants:* Avoiding stimulants such as caffeine and electronics before bedtime promotes a tranquil transition to sleep. We explore how these factors impact the quality of your rest.
*Optimizing Sleep Environment:* Your bedroom should be a sanctuary for sleep. Discussing factors like room temperature, lighting, and mattress quality, we guide you in creating an optimal sleep environment.

**Key Takeaways:**
1. *Sleep as a Reset Button:* Understand the rejuvenating power of sleep as it revitalizes your body and mind.
2. *Consistency Matters:* Appreciate the importance of maintaining a regular sleep schedule for better sleep quality.
3. *Creating Tranquil Nights:* Implement calming bedtime rituals and optimize your sleep environment for a restful night.

**Next Steps:** As we unfold the mysteries of sleep, consider how incorporating these insights into your nightly routine can lead to transformative changes in your overall health. Turn the page and embark on a journey to unlock the rejuvenating potential of quality sleep.

## Quality Sleep Habits: Unleashing the Power of Restorative Slumber

*Introduction:* Quality sleep is not just about the quantity of hours spent in bed; it's about the restorative nature of those hours. In this section, we explore the science behind achieving quality sleep and how cultivating specific habits can enhance the rejuvenating effects of your nightly rest.

**Optimal Sleep Duration:** *Understanding Individual Needs:* While the recommended amount of sleep for adults is 7-9 hours, individual variations exist. We discuss factors that influence your unique sleep requirements.

*Consistency vs. Weekends:* Consistency in sleep patterns, even on weekends, supports your body's natural circadian rhythm and contributes to better overall sleep quality.

**Sleep Environment Optimization:** *Cool, Dark, and Quiet:* A sleep-conducive environment involves optimizing temperature, reducing light exposure, and minimizing noise. Learn how these elements contribute to a comfortable and peaceful sleep space.

*Bedding Essentials:* The right mattress and pillows play a crucial role in supporting proper spinal alignment and ensuring a comfortable night's sleep. We guide you in choosing bedding that suits your needs.

**Limiting Screen Time Before Bed:** *Blue Light Impact:* The blue light emitted by screens can interfere with melatonin production, disrupting your sleep-wake cycle. Discover strategies to minimize screen time before bedtime.

*Establishing Tech-Free Zones:* Creating designated areas in your home free from electronic devices contributes to a more peaceful pre-sleep routine. We discuss the importance of setting boundaries.

**Key Takeaways:**
1. *Personalized Sleep Duration:* Acknowledge the variability in sleep needs and tailor your routine accordingly.
2. *Creating a Sleep Sanctuary:* Understand the significance of an optimized sleep environment for quality rest.
3. *Digital Detox Before Bed:* Limiting screen time and establishing tech-free zones contribute to a more restful night.

**Next Steps:** Now equipped with insights into optimizing the duration and quality of your sleep, consider how these habits align with your current routine. The journey to quality sleep begins with small, intentional steps. Turn the page and let's explore the transformative impact of cultivating these quality sleep habits.

## Exercise as a Pillar of Well-being: Energizing Your Body and Mind

*Introduction:* Exercise is not just a physical activity; it's a cornerstone of holistic well-being. In this section, we unravel the profound benefits of regular exercise, exploring how it positively influences your physical health, mental resilience, and overall quality of life.

**Benefits of Daily Exercise:** *Physical Health:* From cardiovascular fitness to enhanced immune function, we delve into the myriad ways exercise strengthens your body.

*Mental Well-being:* Explore the release of endorphins, often referred to as "feel-good" hormones, and the positive impact of exercise on stress reduction and mental clarity.

**Types of Exercise: Cardio, Strength, Flexibility:** *Cardiovascular Exercise:* Understand the importance of activities that elevate your heart rate, such as running, cycling, or swimming.

*Strength Training:* Explore the benefits of building muscle mass, boosting metabolism, and supporting joint health through strength training exercises.

*Flexibility and Mobility:* Incorporating activities like yoga or stretching routines fosters flexibility, balance, and overall joint health.

**Incorporating Physical Activity into Daily Life:** *Making it Accessible:* Exercise doesn't require a gym membership. Discover simple ways to infuse physical activity into your daily routine, whether at home, work, or outdoors.

*Consistency Over Intensity:* Emphasize the significance of regular, moderate exercise over sporadic intense workouts. Consistency is key to reaping the long-term benefits.

**Key Takeaways:**
1. *Comprehensive Health Impact:* Recognize how exercise positively influences both physical and mental well-being.
2. *Diverse Exercise Modalities:* Understand the importance of incorporating cardio, strength, and flexibility exercises into your routine.
3. *Everyday Movement:* Embrace the idea that exercise is not confined to the gym; it's a daily commitment to movement.

**Next Steps:** Armed with the knowledge of exercise's profound impact, consider how you can integrate physical activity into your daily life. The journey to a more active, energized, and resilient you begins with simple, intentional choices. Turn the page and let's explore the transformative power of making exercise a pillar of your well-being.

# Building a Sustainable Exercise Routine: Making Fitness a Lifelong Commitment

*Introduction:* Embarking on a fitness journey isn't just about short-term goals; it's a commitment to long-term well-being. In this section, we explore the principles of building a sustainable exercise routine that aligns with your lifestyle, ensuring consistency and enjoyment.

**Setting Realistic Goals:** *Understanding Your Starting Point:* Realistic goals consider your current fitness level, time constraints, and personal preferences. We discuss the importance of setting achievable milestones.

*Long-Term Vision:* While short-term goals provide motivation, cultivating a vision for your overall well-being helps sustain a lifelong commitment to fitness.

**Finding Activities You Enjoy:** *Exploring Options:* The world of fitness is diverse. From traditional workouts to unconventional activities, discover what resonates with you. Enjoyment is key to long-term adherence.

*Incorporating Variety:* Avoid monotony by incorporating various activities. This not only keeps things interesting but also ensures a balanced approach to fitness.

**Balancing Cardio and Strength Training:** *Cardiovascular Fitness:*

Understand the benefits of cardio for heart health, endurance, and calorie expenditure.
*Strength Training Essentials:* Explore the importance of building lean muscle mass for metabolism, bone health, and overall functional fitness.

**Designing a Well-Rounded Exercise Routine:** *Frequency and Consistency:* Discuss the optimal frequency of workouts and the importance of consistent effort for lasting results.
*Rest and Recovery:* Emphasize the significance of rest days, allowing your body to recover and preventing burnout or injury.

**Key Takeaways:**
1. *Realistic Goal Setting:* Set achievable, personalized fitness goals based on your starting point and long-term vision.
2. *Enjoyment and Variety:* Find activities you genuinely enjoy to ensure sustainability, and incorporate variety to keep things interesting.
3. *Balanced Approach:* Strike a balance between cardio and strength training, designing a well-rounded routine that supports overall health.

**Next Steps:** Armed with insights into sustainable exercise practices, consider how these principles align with your preferences and lifestyle. The journey to a lifelong commitment to fitness begins with thoughtful, adaptable choices. Turn the page and let's explore the transformative power of building a sustainable exercise routine tailored just for you.

# Morning Rituals for a Productive Day: Energizing Your Mind and Body

*Introduction:* The way you start your morning sets the tone for the entire day. In this section, we explore morning rituals that go beyond the rush, helping you establish a positive and productive mindset for the hours ahead.

**The Power of Morning Stretches:** *Awakening Your Body:* Gentle stretches upon waking promote blood flow, flexibility, and alertness. We discuss simple routines that cater to different fitness levels.

*Mind-Body Connection:* Morning stretches not only enhance physical well-being but also establish a connection between your body and mind, fostering a sense of mindfulness.

**Quick Workouts to Energize:** *Efficient Exercise Options:* Discover short, effective workouts that boost energy levels without consuming much time. From brisk walks to bodyweight exercises, we explore options suitable for busy mornings.

*Benefits Beyond Physical Health:* Exercise in the morning contributes to mental clarity, enhanced mood, and increased productivity throughout the day.

# Elevate Your Life: A Guide to Daily Healthy Living Habits

**Mindful Practices for Mental Clarity:** *Breathing Exercises:* Explore simple yet powerful breathing techniques that promote relaxation and mental focus.

*Visualization and Affirmations:* Incorporating positive visualizations and affirmations during your morning routine sets a positive tone for the day, fostering a resilient mindset.

**Key Takeaways:**
1. *Energizing Morning Stretches:* Incorporate gentle stretches to awaken your body and promote flexibility.
2. *Efficient Workouts:* Explore quick exercise routines to boost energy levels and enhance mental clarity.
3. *Mindful Practices:* Embrace breathing exercises, visualization, and affirmations for a positive and focused mindset.

**Next Steps:** Consider how these morning rituals align with your schedule and preferences. The journey to a more productive day begins with intentional choices in the morning. Turn the page and let's explore the transformative impact of incorporating these energizing morning rituals into your daily routine.

## Nutrition for Energy and Vitality: Fueling Your Body for Optimal Performance

*Introduction:* Nutrition isn't just about satisfying hunger; it's about providing your body with the essential elements it needs to thrive. In this section, we explore the role of balanced nutrition in sustaining energy levels, promoting vitality, and supporting overall health.

**Balanced Diet Essentials:** *Macro and Micronutrients:* Understand the importance of a well-balanced diet that includes carbohydrates, proteins, fats, vitamins, and minerals.

*Whole Foods Approach:* Emphasize the significance of incorporating whole, nutrient-dense foods into your diet. Explore the benefits of a colorful plate filled with a variety of fruits, vegetables, lean proteins, and whole grains.

**Importance of Hydration:** *Hydrating Your Body:* Discuss the critical role of water in maintaining bodily functions. Learn about optimal daily water intake and the impact of dehydration on energy levels.

*Beverage Choices:* Explore alternatives to sugary drinks and caffeinated beverages, prioritizing water, herbal teas, and other hydrating options.

# Elevate Your Life: A Guide to Daily Healthy Living Habits

**Healthy Snacking Habits:** *Smart Snack Choices:* Discover nutritious snack options that provide sustained energy between meals. From fresh fruits to nuts and yogurt, we explore snacks that balance taste and health.

*Portion Control:* Emphasize the importance of mindful eating, including appropriate portion sizes to avoid overconsumption.

**Key Takeaways:**
1. *Nutrient-Dense Eating:* Prioritize a balanced diet rich in a variety of nutrients for optimal health.
2. *Hydration Essentials:* Understand the importance of staying adequately hydrated throughout the day.
3. *Smart Snacking:* Choose nutritious snacks and practice portion control for sustained energy.

**Next Steps:** Consider how these nutrition principles align with your current eating habits. The journey to sustained energy and vitality begins with mindful choices in your daily meals. Turn the page and let's explore the transformative power of adopting a nutritionally rich and balanced lifestyle.

# The Power of Power Naps: Recharge Your Mind in Minutes

*Introduction:* In the quest for productivity and well-being, the power nap stands out as a simple yet potent tool. In this section, we explore the benefits of short daytime naps, uncovering their impact on alertness, creativity, and overall cognitive function.

**Benefits of Short Daytime Naps:** *Enhanced Alertness:* Understand how a brief nap can provide a quick boost in alertness and cognitive performance, making it an effective remedy for the post-lunch dip in energy.

*Mood Improvement:* Explore how power naps contribute to a positive mood by reducing feelings of fatigue and enhancing emotional well-being.

**Ideal Nap Duration and Timing:** *The Goldilocks Zone:* Discover the optimal duration for a power nap, balancing the benefits of improved alertness without experiencing sleep inertia.

*Strategic Timing:* Explore the best times to take a power nap to align with your circadian rhythm, maximizing its effectiveness.

**Creating a Nap-Friendly Environment:** *Quiet and Dark Spaces:* Discuss the importance of finding a conducive environment for napping, emphasizing the role of reduced noise and light.

*Setting Boundaries:* Address concerns related to potential disruption and societal expectations, promoting a culture that recognizes the value of short naps.

**Key Takeaways:**
1. *Quick Boost in Alertness:* Harness the power of short naps for improved cognitive performance.
2. *Mood Enhancement:* Understand how power naps can positively impact mood and emotional well-being.
3. *Strategic Napping:* Learn about the ideal duration and timing of power naps for maximum effectiveness.

**Next Steps:** Consider how incorporating power naps aligns with your daily routine. The journey to enhanced alertness and improved mood begins with a willingness to embrace short moments of rest. Turn the page and let's explore the transformative impact of integrating power naps into your daily life.

## Nutrition for Energy and Vitality: Fueling Your Body for Optimal Performance

*Introduction:* Nutrition serves as the foundation for a vibrant and energetic life. In this section, we delve into the intricacies of dietary choices, exploring how the right nutrients can elevate your energy levels, support vitality, and contribute to overall well-being.

**Balanced Diet Essentials:** *Macronutrients: Carbohydrates, Proteins, Fats:* Recognize the importance of a well-balanced diet that includes carbohydrates for energy, proteins for muscle repair, and healthy fats for various bodily functions.

*Micronutrients: Vitamins and Minerals:* Explore the role of vitamins and minerals in supporting immune function, maintaining bone health, and facilitating various biochemical processes in the body.

**Whole Foods Approach:** *Colorful Plate Philosophy:* Adopt a whole foods approach, filling your plate with a variety of colorful fruits, vegetables, lean proteins, and whole grains. This not only provides essential nutrients but also supports digestive health.

*Minimizing Processed Foods:* Understand the impact of processed foods on energy levels and vitality, and explore alternatives that prioritize natural, nutrient-dense options.

# Elevate Your Life: A Guide to Daily Healthy Living Habits

**Importance of Hydration:** *Hydration and Energy:* Delve into the connection between proper hydration and sustained energy levels. Learn about the signs of dehydration and strategies for maintaining adequate fluid intake.

*Beverage Choices:* Consider the impact of beverage choices, emphasizing water, herbal teas, and other hydrating options over sugary or caffeinated drinks.

**Healthy Snacking Habits:** *Strategic Snacking:* Recognize the role of healthy snacks in maintaining steady energy throughout the day. Explore options like nuts, fruits, and yogurt that balance taste and nutritional value.

*Mindful Eating and Portion Control:* Emphasize the importance of mindful eating, including paying attention to portion sizes to avoid overeating.

**Key Takeaways:**
1. *Nutrient-Rich Diet:* Prioritize a balanced intake of macronutrients and micronutrients for optimal health and vitality.
2. *Whole Foods Prioritization:* Adopt a whole foods approach, minimizing processed foods in favor of natural, nutrient-dense options.
3. *Hydration for Energy:* Understand the vital connection between proper hydration and sustained energy levels.

**Next Steps:** Reflect on your current dietary habits and consider how these nutrition principles align with your lifestyle. The journey to sustained energy and vitality begins with intentional choices in your daily meals. Turn the page and let's explore the transformative power of adopting a nutritionally rich and balanced lifestyle.

## Mindful Eating Practices: Savoring Every Bite for Optimal Well-being

*Introduction:* Mindful eating isn't just about what you consume; it's a holistic approach that involves paying attention to every aspect of your eating experience. In this section, we explore the transformative power of mindfulness in fostering a healthy relationship with food and optimizing your overall well-being.

**Eating with Awareness:** *Present-Moment Focus:* Understand the concept of being fully present during meals. Explore how mindfulness can enhance your appreciation for the sensory aspects of eating.

*Savoring Each Bite:* Embrace the practice of savoring flavors, textures, and aromas. Learn how this simple act can lead to a more enjoyable and satisfying dining experience.

**Portion Control:** *Listening to Hunger and Fullness Cues:* Tune in to your body's signals for hunger and fullness. Explore strategies to avoid overeating, such as eating slowly and recognizing when you're satisfied.

*Balancing Nutrient Intake:* Consider the nutritional composition of your meals and snacks. Mindful eating involves making conscious choices about the quality and quantity of the food you consume.

**The Role of Mindfulness in Healthy Eating:** *Emotional Eating Awareness:* Explore the connection between emotions and eating habits. Mindful eating encourages awareness of emotional triggers and finding alternative ways to cope.

*Breaking Unhealthy Eating Habits:* Identify and address mindless or automatic eating behaviors. Cultivate mindfulness to break free from patterns like emotional eating or snacking out of boredom.

**Key Takeaways:**
1. *Present-Moment Awareness:* Embrace mindful eating practices to fully engage with the sensory experience of each meal.
2. *Portion Control and Balance:* Listen to your body's cues and make conscious choices about portion sizes and nutritional balance.
3. *Mindful Eating for Emotional Well-being:* Use mindfulness to address emotional triggers and break unhealthy eating habits.

**Next Steps:** Reflect on your current eating habits and consider how incorporating mindful practices aligns with your lifestyle. The journey to mindful eating begins with small, intentional steps toward fostering a healthier and more conscious relationship with food. Turn the page and let's explore the transformative impact of mindful eating practices on your overall well-being.

## Stress Management Techniques: Cultivating Calm in the Midst of Chaos

*Introduction:* Stress is an inevitable part of life, but how you manage it can significantly impact your overall well-being. In this section, we explore a variety of stress management techniques designed to help you navigate challenges with resilience, foster emotional balance, and cultivate a sense of calm.

**Identifying Stressors:** *Self-Reflection:* Engage in self-awareness to identify specific stressors in your life. Recognizing the sources of stress is the first step toward effective management.

*External and Internal Stressors:* Distinguish between external stressors (work, relationships) and internal stressors (negative thoughts, self-criticism). Understanding both allows for targeted interventions.

**Relaxation Techniques: Meditation, Deep Breathing:** *Meditation Practices:* Explore mindfulness meditation as a tool to calm the mind, increase self-awareness, and reduce the physiological effects of stress.

*Deep Breathing Exercises:* Understand the power of intentional breathing in activating the body's relaxation response. Practice deep-breathing exercises to alleviate tension and promote a sense of calm.

**Creating a Stress-Free Environment:** *Organizational Strategies:* Implement organization and time management techniques to reduce external stressors. A well-organized environment can contribute to a more relaxed mindset.

*Decluttering Physical and Mental Space:* Recognize the impact of a cluttered space on mental well-being. Explore decluttering practices to create a harmonious living and working environment.

**Key Takeaways:**
1. *Stress Identification:* Reflect on and identify both external and internal stressors in your life.
2. *Mindfulness and Relaxation:* Practice mindfulness meditation and deep breathing exercises to manage stress effectively.
3. *Environment Optimization:* Organize your physical and mental space to create a stress-free environment.

**Next Steps:** Consider how these stress management techniques align with your current lifestyle and stressors. The journey to stress resilience begins with consistent practice and a commitment to your well-being. Turn the page and let's explore the transformative power of incorporating these stress management techniques into your daily life.

## Hygiene and Self-Care: Nurturing Your Body and Mind

*Introduction:* Hygiene and self-care are integral components of overall well-being, contributing to both physical health and mental resilience. In this section, we explore the importance of cultivating healthy hygiene habits and the transformative impact of self-care practices on your holistic health.

**Personal Hygiene Practices:** *Daily Routines:* Establish consistent daily hygiene practices, including bathing, oral care, and skincare. These routines not only maintain physical health but also contribute to a positive self-image.

*Hand Hygiene:* Emphasize the importance of regular handwashing, especially in preventing the spread of illness. Explore proper handwashing techniques and when to prioritize hand hygiene.

**Skincare and Grooming:** *Skin Health:* Discuss the significance of skincare in maintaining healthy skin, preventing issues such as dryness or irritation. Consider a skincare routine tailored to your skin type and needs.

*Grooming Habits:* Understand how grooming practices contribute to overall well-being. From hair care to nail maintenance, grooming habits can boost self-confidence and promote a sense of self-care.

**Mental Health Check-Ins:** *Self-Reflection:* Incorporate mental health check-ins into your routine, reflecting on your emotional state and addressing any stressors or concerns.

*Rest and Relaxation:* Recognize the connection between relaxation and mental well-being. Explore practices such as taking breaks, engaging in hobbies, or enjoying moments of quiet reflection.

**Key Takeaways:**
1. *Consistent Hygiene Routines:* Establish and maintain daily hygiene practices for physical health and a positive self-image.
2. *Skincare and Grooming:* Prioritize skincare and grooming habits to enhance self-confidence and overall well-being.
3. *Mental Health Awareness:* Integrate mental health check-ins and relaxation practices into your routine for emotional well-being.

**Next Steps:** Reflect on your current hygiene and self-care practices and consider how incorporating these habits aligns with your lifestyle. The journey to holistic well-being begins with small, intentional steps toward nurturing both your body and mind. Turn the page and let's explore the transformative power of hygiene and self-care practices in enhancing your overall health and happiness.

# Social Connections and Well-being: Nurturing Relationships for a Fulfilling Life

*Introduction:* Human connection is a fundamental aspect of well-being, influencing not only our emotional state but also our physical health. In this section, we explore the transformative power of social connections, shedding light on the importance of building and maintaining meaningful relationships.

**Understanding the Impact of Social Connections:** *Emotional Support:* Recognize the role of social connections in providing emotional support during challenging times. Strong relationships contribute to resilience and a positive outlook.

*Physical Health Benefits:* Explore the link between social connections and physical health, including reduced stress levels, improved immune function, and a lower risk of chronic diseases.

**Building and Nurturing Relationships:** *Quality Over Quantity:* Emphasize the importance of the quality of relationships over the quantity. Meaningful connections bring more joy and fulfillment than a large but superficial network.

*Investing Time and Effort:* Building and maintaining relationships requires effort and time. Explore strategies for fostering connections, from regular communication to shared activities.

**Family Bonds and Friendships:** *Family Dynamics:* Understand the impact of family relationships on overall well-being. Healthy family dynamics contribute to a supportive and nurturing environment.

*Friendship Dynamics:* Explore the significance of friendships in providing companionship, shared experiences, and a sense of belonging. Cultivate friendships that align with your values and aspirations.

**Virtual Connections and Community:** *Online Communities:* Acknowledge the role of virtual connections in today's interconnected world. Online communities can provide valuable support and a sense of belonging.

*Local Community Engagement:* Get involved in local communities or groups to build connections with those around you. Community engagement enhances a sense of belonging and shared purpose.

**Key Takeaways:**
1. *Emotional Support:* Understand how social connections provide emotional support and contribute to resilience.
2. *Quality Relationships:* Emphasize the importance of quality over quantity in building and maintaining meaningful connections.
3. *Diverse Social Connections:* Cultivate both family bonds and friendships, recognizing the unique contributions each makes to well-being.

**Next Steps:** Reflect on your current social connections and consider how these insights align with your lifestyle. The journey to a more fulfilling life begins with intentional efforts to build and nurture meaningful relationships. Turn the page and let's explore the transformative power of social connections on your overall well-being.

# Technology Detox: Reclaiming Balance in a Digital Age

*Introduction:* In the era of constant connectivity, taking intentional breaks from technology has become essential for overall well-being. In this section, we explore the concept of a technology detox, highlighting its importance in fostering mental clarity, reducing stress, and reclaiming a healthy balance in our digital lives.

**Understanding the Impact of Excessive Screen Time:** *Digital Fatigue:* Recognize the signs of digital fatigue, including eye strain, disrupted sleep patterns, and mental exhaustion. Understand the impact of excessive screen time on overall health.

*Social Comparison and Stress:* Explore the role of social media in contributing to stress and anxiety through constant comparison and curated online personas. Understand the importance of setting healthy boundaries.

**Strategies for a Technology Detox:** *Scheduled Breaks:* Implement scheduled breaks from screens throughout the day. Explore techniques such as the 20-20-20 rule to reduce eye strain and promote a healthier relationship with digital devices.

*Digital Sabbatical:* Consider periodic digital detox days or weekends. Disconnecting from technology allows for a reset, fostering in-person connections and engagement with the physical world.

**Mindful Technology Use:** *Setting Boundaries:* Establish clear boundaries for technology use, both in terms of time spent and the types of activities engaged in. Explore the concept of a digital curfew to promote better sleep.

*Intentional Social Media Use:* Practice mindful and intentional use of social media. Curate your online space to prioritize positive and meaningful content, and consider limiting scrolling time.

**Embracing Offline Activities:** *Reconnecting with Hobbies:* Rediscover offline hobbies and activities that bring joy and fulfillment. Engage in activities that don't involve screens, fostering a balanced and well-rounded lifestyle.

*Quality Face-to-Face Interactions:* Prioritize face-to-face interactions with friends and family. Strengthening in-person connections contributes to a sense of community and belonging.

**Key Takeaways:**
1. *Digital Fatigue Awareness:* Recognize the signs of digital fatigue and the impact of excessive screen time.
2. *Strategies for Detox:* Implement scheduled breaks, periodic digital detox days, and set boundaries for mindful technology use.
3. *Balancing Offline Activities:* Embrace offline hobbies and prioritize face-to-face interactions for a more balanced lifestyle.

**Next Steps:** Reflect on your current technology habits and consider how these insights align with your lifestyle. The journey to a healthier relationship with technology begins with intentional choices to reclaim balance and well-being. Turn the page and let's explore the transformative power of a technology detox in enhancing your overall quality of life.

## Improving Sleep through Lifestyle Choices: Unleashing the Power of Restful Nights

*Introduction:* Quality sleep is not just a result of bedtime habits; it's deeply influenced by lifestyle choices throughout the day. In this section, we explore how various aspects of your daily routine and lifestyle can be optimized to enhance the quality of your sleep, ensuring restful and rejuvenating nights.

**The Role of Lifestyle in Sleep Quality:** *Holistic Sleep Approach:* Recognize that sleep is influenced by various lifestyle factors, including diet, exercise, stress management, and technology use. A holistic approach ensures comprehensive sleep improvement.

*Establishing Consistent Routines:* Understand the importance of consistent wake-up and bedtime routines. Consistency signals your body's internal clock, promoting a more regulated sleep-wake cycle.

**Dietary Choices for Better Sleep:** *Timing of Meals:* Explore the impact of meal timing on sleep. Avoid heavy or large meals close to bedtime, opting for lighter snacks if needed.

*Caffeine and Sleep:* Understand the effects of caffeine on sleep and establish a cut-off time for consumption to prevent interference with your ability to fall asleep.

# Elevate Your Life: A Guide to Daily Healthy Living Habits

**Exercise and Sleep Quality:** *Regular Physical Activity:* Embrace regular exercise as a powerful tool for improving sleep quality. Recognize the importance of timing, with early to midday workouts being most beneficial.

*Avoiding Intense Exercise Before Bed:* Understand the potential disruptive effects of intense exercise close to bedtime. Gentle activities like yoga or stretching are better suited for the evening.

**Stress Management Techniques for Better Sleep:** *Mindfulness Practices:* Engage in mindfulness practices, such as meditation or deep breathing, to manage stress and promote relaxation before bedtime.

*Establishing a Relaxing Bedtime Routine:* Create a calming pre-sleep routine that signals to your body that it's time to wind down. This may include activities like reading, taking a warm bath, or practicing relaxation techniques.

**Optimizing the Sleep Environment:** *Creating a Comfortable Sleep Space:* Explore the importance of a comfortable and conducive sleep environment, including considerations like room temperature, lighting, and the quality of your mattress and pillows.

*Limiting Screen Time Before Bed:* Minimize exposure to screens before bedtime, as the blue light emitted can interfere with melatonin production. Establish a technology-free wind-down period.

**Key Takeaways:**
1. *Holistic Sleep Approach:* Recognize the multifaceted influence of lifestyle choices on sleep quality.
2. *Nutritional Impact:* Consider the timing of meals and the effects of caffeine on sleep.

3. *Exercise Timing:* Embrace regular physical activity but be mindful of the timing, avoiding intense workouts close to bedtime.
4. *Stress Management:* Incorporate mindfulness practices and establish a calming bedtime routine.
5. *Optimizing Sleep Environment:* Create a comfortable sleep space and limit screen time before bed.

**Next Steps:** Reflect on your current lifestyle choices and consider how these insights align with your daily routine. The journey to improved sleep quality begins with intentional adjustments and a commitment to fostering a sleep-friendly lifestyle. Turn the page and let's explore the transformative power of optimizing your daily habits for restful nights.

**Motivation and Accountability: Fanning the Flames of Personal Growth**
*Introduction:* Embarking on a journey of self-improvement requires not only motivation but also a solid foundation of accountability. In this section, we delve into the dynamics of motivation, exploring how to ignite and sustain it, while also establishing mechanisms for accountability to ensure consistent progress towards your goals.

**Understanding Motivation:** *Intrinsic vs. Extrinsic Motivation:* Differentiate between intrinsic motivation, driven by internal factors like passion and personal fulfillment, and extrinsic motivation, influenced by external rewards or pressures. Recognize the power of cultivating intrinsic motivation for lasting commitment.

*Setting Meaningful Goals:* Establish goals that align with your values and aspirations. Meaningful goals serve as powerful motivators, driving sustained effort and enthusiasm.

**Strategies for Sustaining Motivation:** *Visualization Techniques:* Embrace visualization as a tool to imagine the positive outcomes of your efforts. Visualization creates a mental image of success, reinforcing motivation.

*Positive Affirmations:* Practice positive self-talk and affirmations. Cultivate a mindset that supports your journey by acknowledging your capabilities and fostering self-belief.

**Building Accountability Structures:** *Accountability Partners:* Consider enlisting an accountability partner, someone who shares your goals and provides mutual support. Regular check-ins with a partner create a sense of responsibility and encouragement.
*Progress Tracking:* Establish a system for tracking your progress. Whether through journaling, apps, or visual aids, tracking allows you to celebrate successes and identify areas for improvement.

**Overcoming Challenges and Maintaining Consistency:** *Anticipating Setbacks:* Acknowledge that setbacks are a natural part of any journey. Develop resilience by anticipating challenges and formulating strategies to overcome them.
*Creating Rituals and Routines:* Implement rituals and routines that reinforce positive habits. Consistency is key to building momentum and maintaining motivation over the long term.

**Celebrating Milestones:** *Acknowledging Achievements:* Celebrate both small and large achievements along the way. Recognition of progress serves as a powerful motivator, fueling your commitment to the journey.

*Adjusting Goals as Needed:* Be flexible in adjusting goals based on evolving circumstances or aspirations. A dynamic approach ensures that your objectives remain relevant and motivating.

**Key Takeaways:**
1. *Intrinsic Motivation:* Cultivate intrinsic motivation by aligning goals with personal values and passions.

2. *Sustaining Strategies:* Utilize visualization, positive affirmations, and meaningful goal-setting to sustain motivation.
3. *Accountability Structures:* Build accountability through partners, progress tracking, and overcoming challenges.
4. *Consistency and Celebration:* Maintain consistency through rituals, routines, and flexibility. Celebrate achievements to reinforce motivation.

**Next Steps:** Reflect on your current motivations and accountability structures, considering how these insights align with your goals. The journey to personal growth and achievement begins with intentional strategies for sustained motivation and accountability. Turn the page and let's explore the transformative power of these principles in your journey of self-improvement.

# Conclusion: Cultivating a Life of Holistic Well-being

Congratulations on completing this exploration of daily habits that contribute to a life of holistic well-being. As you've journeyed through the pages of this guide, you've encountered a diverse array of practices aimed at nourishing your body, mind, and spirit. Let's recap the key themes and takeaways that can serve as pillars for your ongoing pursuit of a fulfilling and balanced life.

1. **Quality Sleep Habits:**
   - Acknowledge the individuality of sleep needs and cultivate personalized sleep routines.
   - Optimize your sleep environment for comfort, darkness, and quiet.
   - Limit screen time before bedtime and establish tech-free zones in your home.

2. **Exercise as a Pillar of Well-being:**
   - Recognize the comprehensive impact of exercise on physical and mental health.
   - Incorporate diverse modalities, including cardiovascular, strength, and flexibility exercises.
   - Prioritize consistency over intensity in your exercise routine.

3. **Building a Sustainable Exercise Routine:**
   - Set realistic, achievable fitness goals based on your starting point and long-term vision.

- Find activities you genuinely enjoy to ensure sustainability.
- Strike a balance between cardio and strength training for a well-rounded routine.

4. **Morning Rituals for a Productive Day:**
   - Energize your mind and body with morning stretches and quick workouts.
   - Embrace mindful practices like breathing exercises, visualization, and affirmations.
   - Cultivate a positive mindset with intentional morning rituals.

5. **Nutrition for Energy and Vitality:**
   - Prioritize a balanced diet rich in macro and micronutrients through whole foods.
   - Stay adequately hydrated with water and hydrating beverages.
   - Choose smart snacks and practice mindful eating for sustained energy.

6. **The Power of Power Naps:**
   - Harness the benefits of short daytime naps for improved alertness and mood.
   - Understand the ideal duration and timing of power naps.
   - Create a nap-friendly environment for quick rejuvenation.

7. **Mindful Eating Practices:**
   - Embrace mindfulness in your eating habits to savor and appreciate each bite.
   - Pay attention to hunger and fullness cues, practicing portion control.
   - Address emotional eating through self-reflection and breaking unhealthy habits.

8. **Stress Management Techniques:**
   - Identify stressors and distinguish between external and internal stressors.

- Engage in relaxation techniques, including meditation and deep breathing.
- Optimize your environment for stress reduction through organization and decluttering.

9. **Hygiene and Self-Care:**
   - Establish consistent personal hygiene routines for physical health and positive self-image.
   - Prioritize skincare, grooming, and mental health check-ins.
   - Cultivate a holistic approach to hygiene that nurtures both body and mind.

10. **Social Connections and Well-being:**
    - Recognize the emotional and physical health benefits of strong social connections.
    - Build and nurture meaningful relationships with both family and friends.
    - Engage in both virtual and local communities for a sense of belonging.

11. **Technology Detox:**
    - Understand the impact of excessive screen time on physical and mental health.
    - Implement strategies for a technology detox, including scheduled breaks and digital sabbaticals.
    - Embrace offline activities and create boundaries for mindful technology use.

12. **Improving Sleep through Lifestyle Choices:**
    - Adopt a holistic approach to sleep by considering diet, exercise, stress management, and technology use.
    - Cultivate consistent wake-up and bedtime routines for a regulated sleep-wake cycle.
    - Optimize your sleep environment and limit screen time before bedtime.

13. **Motivation and Accountability:**
    - Cultivate intrinsic motivation aligned with your values and passions.

- Sustain motivation through visualization, positive affirmations, and meaningful goal-setting.
- Build accountability structures with partners, progress tracking, and consistent routines.

In embracing these habits, remember that well-being is a dynamic and ongoing journey. It's about making intentional choices each day that contribute to your overall health and happiness. As you integrate these practices into your life, allow room for flexibility, self-compassion, and adaptation. You have the power to shape your well-being, and this guide serves as a compass for navigating the path toward a more vibrant and fulfilling life.

May your journey be transformative, and may each intentional choice bring you closer to a life of holistic well-being.

# ABOUT THE AUTHOR

Habib Zakari Mohammed
Is a Mechanical Engineer by profession and an avid IT guru. He has been able to master a disciplined healthy lifestyle & thus stayed healthy and fit over the years as outlined in his very first of many books.